MULTIPLE SCLEROSIS COOKBOOK

MEGA BUNDLE – 3 Manuscripts in 1 – 120+ Multiple Sclerosis - friendly recipes including smoothies, pies, and pancakes for a delicious and tasty diet

TABLE OF CONTENTS

3

This document is geared towards providing exact and reliable information in regards to the topic and issue covered. The publication is sold with the idea that the publisher is not required to render accounting, officially permitted, or otherwise, qualified services. If advice is necessary, legal or professional, a practiced individual in the profession should be ordered.

- From a Declaration of Principles which was accepted and approved equally by a Committee of the American Bar Association and a Committee of Publishers and Associations.

Introduction

Multiple Sclerosis recipes for personal enjoyment but also for family enjoyment. You will love them for sure for how easy it is to prepare them.

BREAKFAST

HERB FRITTATA

Serves: *3*

Prep Time: *10*   Minutes

Cook Time: *20*   Minutes

Total Time: *30*   Minutes

INGREDIENTS

- 6 eggs
- 1 tbsp parsley
- some spinach leaves
- ¼ tsp salt
- a pinch pepper

DIRECTIONS

1. Preheat your oven to 350°F
2. Boil the spinach and then remove the water
3. In a bowl, whisk the eggs and add the spinach and the other ingredients
4. Put the mix into the oven for 20 min

GOLDEN PANCAKES

Serves: *4*
Prep Time: *10*   Minutes

Cook Time: *15*   Minutes

Total Time: *25*   Minutes

INGREDIENTS

- a cup almond flour
- 2 cups water
- onion
- a pinch of salt

DIRECTIONS

1. In a bowl, combine the flour with water until it gets consistent
2. Chop the onion and combine it with the mixture
3. Spread your mixture on the frying pan and after 3 minutes, flip it over and there you have it

Serves: 2

Prep Time: 5   Minutes

Cook Time: 10   Minutes

Total Time: 15   Minutes

INGREDIENTS

- a cup quinoa
- a cup almond milk
- a cup water
- a pinch salt
- a sliced fruit

DIRECTIONS

1. Mix all the ingredients in a saucepan
2. After you get it to a boil, cover the top and let it sit until water is absorbed

OATMEAL WITH FRUIT

Serves: *2*
Prep Time: *10*   Minutes

Cook Time: *15*   Minutes

Total Time: *25*   Minutes

INGREDIENTS

- a cup oats
- any fruits you like
- a glass water
- a glass milk
- sweetener or honey

DIRECTIONS

1. Combine the oats with water in a saucepan and let it boil
2. Drain the water and let it sit for 5 minutes and then and the milk
3. Slice your fruits and put them in a frying pan with some water and let them covered for 3 minutes.
4. Mix the oats together with the fruits and you are ready to serve

ROASTED OATMEAL

Serves: *2*

Prep Time: *10*   Minutes

Cook Time: *20*   Minutes

Total Time: *30*   Minutes

INGREDIENTS

- 3 tbsp raw coconut flakes
- 1 tbsp oil
- 1 cup oat flakes
- 1 tsp sugar
- 3 cups water

DIRECTIONS

1. Boil the water and add the oil and sugar
2. Over the boiling water, add the oats and stir until it gets soft and creamy
3. Top it with the coconut flakes and serve

GINGER APPLE SAUCE

Serves: *1*

Prep Time: *10*   Minutes

Cook Time: *5*   Minutes

Total Time: *15*   Minutes

INGREDIENTS

- 1 apple
- 1 tsp dry ginger
- 1 tbsp sugar

DIRECTIONS

1. **In a saucepan add the sliced apple with 1 cup of water and let it boil with the sugar**
2. **Add the ginger and continue stirring**
3. **Served warm**

BANANAS WITH LEMON JUICE AND CILANTRO

Serves: **2**

Prep Time: **5** Minutes

Cook Time: **5** Minutes

Total Time: **10** Minutes

INGREDIENTS

- 2 bananas
- 1 cup fresh cilantro
- 2 tbsp lemon juice

DIRECTIONS

1. Cut the bananas and add the other ingredients and mix them well, but gently and it is ready to be served

SEASONAL BAKED APPLE WITH CINNAMON AND ROSEMARY

Serves: 3
Prep Time: 5 Minutes

Cook Time: 25 Minutes

Total Time: 30 Minutes

INGREDIENTS

- 3 apples
- 1 tsp cinnamon
- little butter
- 1 tsp rosemary

DIRECTIONS

1. Preheat the oven to 370°F
2. Arrange your sliced apples in a baking plate
3. In a pan, melt the butter and pour it over the apples evenly
4. Sprinkle the cinnamon and the rosemary on top of the slices. Put it in the oven for 30-35 minutes

SPRING PANCAKES

Serves: **4**

Prep Time: **10** Minutes

Cook Time: **15** Minutes

Total Time: **25** Minutes

INGREDIENTS

- 1 tbsp vinegar
- 1 tsp chili
- 1 tsp coriander
- 1 tbsp butter
- 1 cup ground corn
- a pinch salt

DIRECTIONS

1. Combine the coriander, chili, and salt in a bowl
2. In a saucepan, boil 1 cup water with salt and vinegar and pour it over the mixture
3. Add the ground corn and knead until it has a uniform texture
4. Create medium sized balls out of the dough and flatten it after your preference
5. Fry the dough in a frying pan with butter and serve it

RICE CREAM WITH GINGER

Serves: **2**

Prep Time: **10**   Minutes

Cook Time: **30**   Minutes

Total Time: **40**   Minutes

INGREDIENTS

- 1 cup rice
- a pinch pepper
- 1 clove garlic
- 1 tbsp butter
- 1 tsp dry ginger
- 1 pinch salt

DIRECTIONS

1. Fry the chopped garlic in a pot with butter and the dry ginger for 3 minutes
2. Add 3 cups water and let it boil
3. While stirring, add the rice and the other ingredients and keep stirring for 5-6 minutes
4. Reduce the heat to minimum and let it drain for 6 minutes

MUSHROOM OMELETTE

Serves: **1**

Prep Time: **5**   Minutes

Cook Time: **10**   Minutes

Total Time: **15**   Minutes

INGREDIENTS

- 2 eggs
- ¼ tsp salt
- ¼ tsp black pepper
- 1 tablespoon olive oil
- ¼ cup cheese
- ¼ tsp basil
- 1 cup mushrooms

DIRECTIONS

1. In a bowl combine all ingredients together and mix well
2. In a skillet heat olive oil and pour the egg mixture
3. Cook for 1-2 minutes per side
4. When ready remove omelette from the skillet and serve

BANANA AND APPLE PANCAKES

Serves: *3*
Prep Time: *5*   Minutes

Cook Time: *5*   Minutes

Total Time: *10*   Minutes

INGREDIENTS

- 1 apple
- 5 eggs
- 2 bananas
- 1 tablespoon coconut oil

DIRECTIONS

1. In a bowl mash the bananas and apples
2. Crack the eggs and mix them all together
3. In a frying pan pour one-two spoons of mixture
4. Cook each pancake for 1-2 minutes per side
5. Remove and serve with honey

Serves: **1**

Prep Time: **5** Minutes

Cook Time: **5** Minutes

Total Time: **10** Minutes

INGREDIENTS

- 3 cups yogurt
- ½ cup almonds
- ¼ cup blueberries
- 1 cup strawberries
- ½ tsp lemon juice

DIRECTIONS

1. In a bowl place all ingredients
2. Mixed well and refrigerate overnight
3. Serve in the morning

Serves: *1*
Prep Time: *5*   Minutes

Cook Time: *5*   Minutes

Total Time: *10*   Minutes

INGREDIENTS

- ¼ cup oats
- ¼ cup milk
- ½ cup yogurt
- 1 tsp vanilla extract
- 1 tsp honey

DIRECTIONS

1. In a bowl combine all ingredients
2. Refrigerate overnight
3. Serve in the morning

Serves:	*2*	
Prep Time:	*10*	Minutes
Cook Time:	*10*	Minutes
Total Time:	*20*	Minutes

INGREDIENTS

- 2 scrambled eggs
- 3 oz. salmon
- ½ avocado

DIRECTIONS

1. Scramble eggs and transfer to a plate
2. Add salmon, avocado slices and serve

BAKED APPLES

Serves: **2**

Prep Time: **10** Minutes

Cook Time: **50** Minutes

Total Time: **60** Minutes

INGREDIENTS

- ½ tsp cinnamon
- 1 tsp canola oil
- 1 tablespoon oats
- 1 tsp sugar
- 2 apples

DIRECTIONS

1. Preheat the oven to 325 F
2. In a bowl mix sugar, cinnamon, oats and oil
3. Stuff into cored apples and bake for 40-50 minutes
4. Remove and serve

GREEK OMELET

Serves:	**2**	
Prep Time:	**5**	Minutes
Cook Time:	**10**	Minutes
Total Time:	**15**	Minutes

INGREDIENTS

- 3 eggs
- ½ cup parsley
- ¼ tsp salt
- ¼ tsp ground pepper
- 1 tsp olive oil
- ¼ cup spinach
- 1 plum tomato
- ½ cup feta cheese
- 6 pitted Kalamata olives

DIRECTIONS

1. In a bowl whisk together eggs, parsley, pepper and salt
2. In a skillet add egg mixture and sprinkle remaining ingredients
3. Cook for 2-3 minutes per side
4. When ready, remove and serve

FRENCH TOAST

Serves: **2**

Prep Time: **10** Minutes

Cook Time: **10** Minutes

Total Time: **20** Minutes

INGREDIENTS

- ½ cup peanut butter
- 2 bread slices
- 2 eggs
- ¼ cup almond milk
- 1 tsp vanilla extract
- 1 tablespoon sugar

DIRECTIONS

1. In a bowl whisk together eggs, vanilla extract, sugar and almond milk
2. Spread peanut butter over bread slices and top with bread slices
3. Dip each sandwich in egg mixture
4. Place sandwiches in a pan and cook for 5-6 minutes per side or until golden brown
5. When ready, remove and serve

SCRAMBLED EGGS

Serves: **1**

Prep Time: **10** Minutes

Cook Time: **10** Minutes

Total Time: **20** Minutes

INGREDIENTS

- 6 eggs
- ½ cup low fat milk
- ¼ tsp salt
- ¼ tsp pepper
- 1 tablespoon butter
- ½ cup cream cheese
- ½ cup Parmesan cheese

DIRECTIONS

1. In a bowl whisk together eggs, salt, milk and pepper
2. In a skillet pour egg mixture and sprinkle cream cheese and cook for 2-3 minutes per side
3. Remove and serve with parmesan cheese

EASY SUNDAY MORNING BAKED EGGS

Serves: 2

Prep Time: 5   Minutes

Cook Time: 25   Minutes

Total Time: *30*   Minutes

INGREDIENTS

- 2 Tsp butter
- ¼ shredded red cabbage
- 5 eggs
- ¼ Tsp black pepper
- 1 Tsp grated Parmesan cheese
- 6 cherry tomatoes
- 7 basil leaves

DIRECTIONS

1. Preheat the oven to 400F
2. Divide the butter and place it in the oven until is melted.
3. Sprinkle the cabbage, basil and the tomatoes and crack two eggs into the ramekins.
4. Bake to the desired level of doneness.
5. Sprinkle with Parmesan cheese and black pepper.

RATATOUILLE HASH UNDER FRIED EGGS

Serves: 2

Prep Time: 15   Minutes

Cook Time: 35   Minutes

Total Time: 50   Minutes

INGREDIENTS

- 2 ounces red bell pepper
- 1/8 Tsp salt
- 1/3 cup scallion greens
- 2-ounces zucchini
- ¾ Tsp oregano
- 2-ounces eggplant
- 3 eggs
- 4 Tsp olive oil
- ½ lbs. red potatoes
- 1/8 Tsp black pepper

DIRECTIONS

1. In a skillet heat 2 teaspoons of garlic oil over over medium heat
2. Add potatoes and cook until golden brown for 2-3 minutes
3. Sauté and stir for 1-2 minutes, add eggplant, pepper and salt
4. Cook the vegetables until they are soft for 5 minutes

5. Add oregano, zucchini and cook for 4-5 minutes, add water and stir
6. Remove from heat and stir in the scallions
7. Heat a frying pan and add 1 teaspoon of garlic oil
8. Add eggs into skillet and salt, cook until eggs are ready

COCONUT RASPEBERRY OATMEAL

Serves: *1*

Prep Time: *15*   Minutes

Cook Time: *10*   Minutes

Total Time: *25*   Minutes

INGREDIENTS

- ¼ cup oats
- ¾ cup coconut milk
- 2 tablespoons coconut flakes
- 2 teaspoons chia seeds
- ½ cup raspberries

DIRECTIONS

1. In a pot whisk oat, coconut milk, salt, raspberries over medium heat
2. Simmer for 10 minutes until oats are tender and add water
3. Pour oatmeal into a bowl with coconut flakes

PECAN BROWN BUTTER OAT

Serves: **10**

Prep Time: **15**   Minutes

Cook Time: **30**   Minutes

Total Time: **45**   Minutes

INGREDIENTS

- ½ cup pecan halves
- ½ cup butter
- 1/8 teaspoon salt
- 2 teaspoon vanilla extract
- 2 ½ cups rolled oats
- ¼ cup corn syrup
- ½ cup packed brown sugar

DIRECTIONS

1. Preheat oven to 325 F and line a baking dish with parchment
2. Place pecans on a baking sheet and toast for 5-10 minutes
3. Remove from oven and pour in a bowl
4. In a saucepan melt butter over medium heat for 4-5 minutes
5. Stir in brown sugar salt and boil for 1-2 minutes
6. Add oats and pecans to the saucepan and stir, pour the mixture in the baking dish, bake for 15-20 minutes
7. Remove from the oven and let it cook for 10-15 minutes

SPINACH AND QUINOA BREAKFAST

Serves: *8*

Prep Time: **25**   Minutes

Cook Time: **25**   Minutes

Total Time: *50*   Minutes

INGREDIENTS

- 1/3 cup quinoa
- 2/3 cup water
- 1/16 teaspoon black pepper
- 2 tablespoons scallion
- 1 ½ ounces bacon
- 4-ounces spinach
- 5 large eggs
- ¼ teaspoon thyme leaves
- 2 pinches sage
- ¼ teaspoon salt
- 2 cups cheddar cheese

DIRECTIONS

1. Preheat oven to 325 F
2. In a saucepan combine quinoa and water and let them boil, after 10-15 minutes remove from heat

3. In a microwave place the frozen spinach and cook for 2-3 minutes

4. In a bowl whisk the eggs and add salt, pepper, scallions, sage and mix with quinoa, bacon and cheese

5. Grease 10 cups of a muffin tin with baking spray and divide the mixture, bake for 20-25 minutes

6. Remove from the oven and let cool them cool before serving

MORNING SAUSAGE

Serves: *4*

Prep Time: *10*   Minutes

Cook Time: *10*   Minutes

Total Time: *10*   Minutes

INGREDIENTS

- 1 lb. ground turkey
- 1 tsp sage
- ½ tsp. salt
- ¼ tsp garlic
- dash white pepper
- dash cayenne pepper
- dash ground nutmeg

DIRECTIONS

1. In a bowl mix all ingredients together
2. Form into patties and cook for 2-3 minutes per side or until golden brown
3. Remove and serve

SAUSAGE BREAKFAST SANDWICH

Serves: 2

Prep Time: 5   Minutes

Cook Time: 15   Minutes

Total Time: 20   Minutes

INGREDIENTS

- ¼ cup egg substitute
- 1 muffin
- 1 turkey sausage patty
- 1 tablespoon cheddar cheese

DIRECTIONS

1. In a skillet pour egg and cook on low heat
2. Place turkey sausage patty in a pan and cook for 4-5 minutes per side
3. On a toasted muffin place the cooked egg, top with a sausage patty and cheddar cheese
4. Serve when ready

BREAKFAST GRANOLA

Serves: 2

Prep Time: 5   Minutes

Cook Time: 30   Minutes

Total Time: 35   Minutes

INGREDIENTS

- 1 tsp vanilla extract
- 1 tablespoon honey
- 1 lb. rolled oats
- 2 tablespoons sesame seeds
- ¼ lb. almonds
- ¼ lb. berries

DIRECTIONS

1. Preheat the oven to 325 F
2. Spread the granola onto a baking sheet
3. Bake for 12-15 minutes, remove and mix everything
4. Bake for another 12-15 minutes or until slightly brown
5. When ready remove from the oven and serve

PANCAKES

BANANA PANCAKES

Serves: **4**

Prep Time: **10**   Minutes

Cook Time: **20**   Minutes

Total Time: **30**   Minutes

INGREDIENTS

- 1 cup whole wheat flour
- ¼ tsp baking soda
- ¼ tsp baking powder
- 1 cup mashed banana
- 2 eggs
- 1 cup milk

DIRECTIONS

1. In a bowl combine all ingredients together and mix well
2. In a skillet heat olive oil
3. Pour ¼ of the batter and cook each pancake for 1-2 minutes per side
4. When ready remove from heat and serve

COOKIES

BREAKFAST COOKIES

Serves: **8-12**

Prep Time: **5**   Minutes

Cook Time: **15**   Minutes

Total Time: **20**   Minutes

INGREDIENTS

- 1 cup rolled oats
- ¼ cup applesauce
- ½ tsp vanilla extract
- 3 tablespoons chocolate chips
- 2 tablespoons dried fruits
- 1 tsp cinnamon

DIRECTIONS

1. Preheat the oven to 325 F
2. In a bowl combine all ingredients together and mix well
3. Scoop cookies using an ice cream scoop
4. Place cookies onto a prepared baking sheet
5. Place in the oven for 12-15 minutes or until the cookies are done
6. When ready remove from the oven and serve

PINK SMOOTHIE

Serves: *1*
Prep Time: 5   Minutes
Cook Time: 5   Minutes
Total Time: *10* Minutes

INGREDIENTS

- 2 bananas
- ½ cup dragon fruit
- 1 tsp coconut flakes
- 1 tsp coconut flakes
- 1 cup coconut water

DIRECTIONS

1. In a blender place all ingredients and blend until smooth
2. Pour smoothie in a glass and serve

APPLE BANANA SMOOTHIE

Serves: **1**

Prep Time: 5 Minutes

Cook Time: 5 Minutes

Total Time: **10** Minutes

INGREDIENTS

- 1 banana
- 1 apple
- 3 tablespoons peanut butter
- ¼ cup almonds
- 1 cup ice

DIRECTIONS

1. In a blender place all ingredients and blend until smooth
2. Pour smoothie in a glass and serve

CARDAMOM SMOOTHIE

Serves: *1*

Prep Time: 5   Minutes

Cook Time: 5   Minutes

Total Time: *10*   Minutes

INGREDIENTS

- 1 beetroot
- 1 cup coconut milk
- 1 banana
- 2 cardamom seeds
- 1 cup ice
- 1 tsp vanilla extract
- 1 tsp lemon juice

DIRECTIONS

1. In a blender place all ingredients and blend until smooth
2. Pour smoothie in a glass and serve

VEGAN SMOOTHIE

Serves: *1*

Prep Time: *5*   Minutes

Cook Time: *5*   Minutes

Total Time: *10* Minutes

INGREDIENTS

- 1 banana
- 2 tablespoons oats
- 2 tsp nut butter
- 2 tsp pumpkin puree
- 1 cup soy milk

DIRECTIONS

1. In a blender place all ingredients and blend until smooth
2. Pour smoothie in a glass and serve

BLACKBERRY SMOOTHIE

Serves: *1*

Prep Time: 5   Minutes

Cook Time: 5   Minutes

Total Time: *10*   Minutes

INGREDIENTS

- 1 lb. berries
- 1 apple
- 1 cup coconut milk
- ¼ cup vanilla yogurt
- 2 oz. oats

DIRECTIONS

1. In a blender place all ingredients and blend until smooth
2. Pour smoothie in a glass and serve

STRAWBERRY SMOOTHIE

Serves: **1**

Prep Time: **5**   Minutes

Cook Time: **5**   Minutes

Total Time: **10** Minutes

INGREDIENTS

- 1 lb. strawberries
- ½ cup vanilla yogurt
- 1 tsp brown sugar
- 1 cup ice

DIRECTIONS

1. **In a blender place all ingredients and blend until smooth**
2. **Pour smoothie in a glass and serve**

MANGO SMOOTHIE

Serves: *1*

Prep Time: 5   Minutes

Cook Time: 5   Minutes

Total Time: *10*   Minutes

INGREDIENTS

- 1 mango
- 1 banana
- 1 cup vanilla yogurt
- 1 cup ice

DIRECTIONS

1. In a blender place all ingredients and blend until smooth
2. Pour smoothie in a glass and serve

BANANA SMOOTHIE

Serves: *1*

Prep Time: *5*   Minutes

Cook Time: *5*   Minutes

Total Time: *10*   Minutes

INGREDIENTS

- 1 cup vanilla yogurt
- 1 banana
- 1 cup skimmed milk
- 1 tsp cinnamon

DIRECTIONS

1. In a blender place all ingredients and blend until smooth
2. Pour smoothie in a glass and serve

MUFFINS

SIMPLE MUFFINS

Serves: **8-12**

Prep Time: **10**   Minutes

Cook Time: **20**   Minutes

Total Time: **30**   Minutes

INGREDIENTS

- 2 eggs
- 1 tablespoon olive oil
- 1 cup milk
- 2 cups whole wheat flour
- 1 tsp baking soda
- ¼ tsp baking soda
- 1 cup pumpkin puree
- 1 tsp cinnamon
- ¼ cup molasses

DIRECTIONS

1. In a bowl combine all dry ingredients
2. In another bowl combine all dry ingredients
3. Combine wet and dry ingredients together
4. Pour mixture into 8-12 prepared muffin cups, fill 2/3 of the cups

5. Bake for 18-20 minutes at 375 F
6. When ready remove from the oven and serve

ORANGE MUFFINS

Serves: **6**

Prep Time: **10** Minutes

Cook Time: **20** Minutes

Total Time: **30** Minutes

INGREDIENTS

- 1 cup flour
- ¼ cup sugar
- 1 tsp baking powder
- ¼ tsp salt
- 2 eggs
- ¼ cup almond milk
- ½ cup butter
- 1 tsp grated orange rind

DIRECTIONS

1. Preheat oven to 375 F
2. In a bowl mix flour, sugar, salt and baking powder
3. Stir together almond, butter, eggs and dry ingredients and mix well
4. Spoon batter into muffin cups and bake for 18-20 ur until golden brown, remove and serve

BLUEBERRY MUFFINS

Serves: **4**

Prep Time: **10**   Minutes

Cook Time: **20**   Minutes

Total Time: **30**   Minutes

INGREDIENTS

- 2 cups flour
- ½ cup sugar
- 1 tablespoon baking powder
- ¼ tsp salt
- 1 cup almond milk
- ½ cup butter
- 1 egg
- 1 cup blueberries
- 1 cup powdered sugar
- 1 tablespoon lemon juice

DIRECTIONS

1. Preheat the oven to 375 F
2. In a bowl place baking powder, salt, milk, butter and mix well
3. Stir together butter, milk and egg and mix well
4. Add dry ingredients, berries and mix again

5. Spoon batter into muffin cuts and bake for 18-20 minutes or until golden brown

6. When ready, remove and serve

SECOND COOKBOOK

BREAKFAST RECIPES

EGG MUFFINS WITH CHEESE

Serves: **4**

Prep Time: **10** Minutes

Cook Time: **20** Minutes

Total Time: **30** Minutes

INGREDIENTS

- ¼ cup red pepper
- ¼ zucchini
- 1 tablespoon jalapeno
- 6 eggs
- 1 cup cheddar cheese
- ¼ tsp salt
- ¼ cup red onions

DIRECTIONS

1. Preheat oven to 375 F and place 6 baking cups inside muffin tin
2. In a bowl mix zucchini, cheese, eggs, salt, pepper ad jalapeno
3. Divide the mixture between you baking cups and bake for 15-20 minutes

BLUEBERRY MUFFINS

Serves: **8**

Prep Time: **10** Minutes

Cook Time: **30** Minutes

Total Time: **40** Minutes

INGREDIENTS

- **2 cups almond flour**
- **2 eggs**
- **½ tsp cream tartar**
- **¼ tsp baking soda**
- **¼ tsp salt**
- **1 cup blueberries**
- **¼ tsp vanilla extract**
- **½ cup arrowroot flour**
- **½ cup maple syrup**

DIRECTIONS

1. **Preheat oven to 325 F**
2. **In a bowl mix all the flour ingredients, salt and baking soda**
3. **Add maple syrup, vanilla extract, eggs and stir**
4. **Add blueberries and pour over parchment paper and bake for 20 minutes**

LEMON MUFFINS

Serves: *8*

Prep Time: *15* Minutes

Cook Time: *30* Minutes

Total Time: *45* Minutes

INGREDIENTS

- 2 cups almond flour
- ¼ tsp salt
- zest of one lemon
- 1 tablespoon poppy seeds
- ¼ baking soda
- 1 tablespoon coconut flour
- 4 eggs
- ¼ cup honey
- 1 tsp sucanat
- ¾ tsp vanilla extract
- 1 tsp lemon extract

DIRECTIONS

1. Preheat oven to 325 F and grease muffin cups with coconut oil
2. In a bowl mix almond and coconut flour, salt, baking soda and poppy seeds
3. In another bowl whisk together lemon extract, zest, eggs, vanilla, honey and pour the mixture into muffin cups
4. Mix almond flour with sucanat and sprinkle over the muffins

5. Bake for 20-25 minutes, remove when ready and serve

FRENCH TOAST

Serves: *2*

Prep Time: *10* Minutes

Cook Time: *40* Minutes

Total Time: *50* Minutes

INGREDIENTS

- ½ cup butter
- ½ cup applesauce
- 1 tablespoon honey
- ¼ tsp salt
- 5 eggs
- ¼ cup coconut flour

DIRECTIONS

1. Preheat oven to 325 F and grease one pan with butter
2. In a bowl mix eggs, salt, honey, apple sauce, coconut flour, salt and pour the batter into the pan
3. Bake for 35-40 minutes until bread is brown
4. Remove the pan and let it cool before serving

QUICHE WITH BACON AND TOMATO

Serves: *4*

Prep Time: *15*   Minutes

Cook Time: *30*   Minutes

Total Time: *45*   Minutes

INGREDIENTS

- 10 eggs
- 6 oz. cheese
- ¼ tsp salt
- ¼ tsp pepper
- 1 potato
- 5 strips of bacon
- ¼ cup green onion
- ¼ cup tomato

DIRECTIONS

1. Preheat oven to 3250 F
2. In a skillet fry bacon for 5-10 minutes and remove when ready
3. In a skillet place potato slices
4. In a bowl whisk eggs, grate cheese and mix with pepper, tomato, onion and salt
5. Pour the mixture into skillet
6. Place the skillet in the oven and bake for 20 minutes

APPLE FRITTER

Serves: **4**

Prep Time: **10** Minutes

Cook Time: **30** Minutes

Total Time: **40** Minutes

INGREDIENTS

- **2 apples**
- **¼ tsp lemon juice**
- **1 tsp cinnamon**
- **1 tablespoon maple sugar**

Dough

- **1 egg**
- **¼ tsp cinnamon**
- **¼ tsp nutmeg**
- **sal**
- **¼ cup arrowroot flour**
- **¼ tsp maple sugar**
- **1 tsp maple syrup**

DIRECTIONS

1. **In a bowl place the apples with cinnamon, maple syrup, lemon juice and coconut sugar**

2. In another bowl mix, nutmeg, cinnamon, salt, maple sugar, arrowroot flour
3. In a skillet heat oil and add the apples to the dough mixture and then place into skillet
4. Cook 2-3 minutes each side each apple slice
5. Remove and serve

BREAKFAST SAUSAGE

Serves: *4*

Prep Time: *10* Minutes

Cook Time: *10* Minutes

Total Time: *20* Minutes

INGREDIENTS

- 1-pound lean pork
- 1 tablespoon maple syrup
- 1 tsp Italian seasoning
- 1 tsp salt
- ¼ tsp thyme

DIRECTIONS

1. In a bowl mix all the ingredients
2. Form into patties and fry in a skillet
3. Remove when golden brown and serve

ALMOND FLOUR PANCAKES

Serves: **4**

Prep Time: **10** Minutes

Cook Time: **20** Minutes

Total Time: **30** Minutes

INGREDIENTS

- 1 cup almond flour
- 1 egg
- 1tsp vanilla extract
- ¼ tsp baking soda
- salt
- ¾ cup milk
- sliced fruits (strawberries, bananas, blueberries)

DIRECTIONS

1. Preheat griddle to 300 F
2. In a bowl whisk together baking soda, salt, almond flour, eggs, milk and vanilla extract
3. Pour the mixture on the griddle and cook each pancake for2-3 minutes per side
4. Remove and serve with fruit and maple syrup on top

BLUEBERRY PANCAKES

Serves: **8**

Prep Time: **10**   Minutes

Cook Time: **10**   Minutes

Total Time: **20**   Minutes

INGREDIENTS

- 1 cups buckwheat flour
- 1 cups water
- ¼ tsp baking soda
- ¼ tsp salt
- 1 cups blueberry
- juice from 2 lemons
- ½ cup tapioca flour
- 1 egg
- ¼ cup avocado oil
- 2 tablespoons cane sugar
- 2 tsp almond extract
- 1 tsp baking powder

DIRECTIONS

1. Make the pancakes mixture the night before cooking
2. In a bowl mix buckwheat flour, lemon juice, water and stir
3. In the morning add the rest of the ingredients in the mixture

4. In a skillet pour the pancakes mixture and cook 2-3 minutes per side

BACON AND EGG BREAKFAST

Serves: *4*

Prep Time: *10* Minutes

Cook Time: *40* Minutes

Total Time: *50* Minutes

INGREDIENTS

- 1 8-ounce bacon package
- 2 eggs
- coconut oil
- mushrooms

DIRECTIONS

1. Preheat oven to 350 F
2. Grease 4 muffin thin and then line the walls of the muffin cup with with a bacon strip, bake for 10-12 minutes
3. In a bowl whisk together the eggs with garlic, tomatoes, cheese, spinach and mushrooms
4. Pour the mixture in the muffin cup and bake for 25-30 minutes
5. When ready remove from the oven and serve

MAPLE GRANOLA

Serves: **4**

Prep Time: **10** Minutes

Cook Time: **30** Minutes

Total Time: **40** Minutes

INGREDIENTS

- 1 cup almond slivers
- ½ tsp salt
- 1 cup coconut flakes
- 5 tablespoons male syrup
- 1 cup sunflower seeds
- 1 cup pecans
- 1 tablespoon vanilla extract
- 1 tsp cinnamon

DIRECTIONS

1. Preheat oven to 300 F and line a baking sheet with parchment paper
2. In a bowl place coconut flakes, pecans, sunflower seeds, almond sliver and mix
3. In another bowl mix vanilla extract, maple syrup, salt and cinnamon
4. Pour the mixture into the pan and bake for 35-40 minutes
5. When ready remove and cut into smaller pieces and serve

GRAIN PORRIDGE

Serves: *4*

Prep Time: *10* Minutes

Cook Time: *50* Minutes

Total Time: *60* Minutes

INGREDIENTS

- 1 cup oats
- ½ cup maple syrup
- 1 tablespoon coconut oil
- ¼ cup currants
- 1 tablespoon fenugreek seeds
- 1 tablespoon fennel seeds
- 1 cup barley
- 1 tsp salt
- 1 cup quinoa
- ½ cup pumpkin seeds
- 1 tablespoon apple cider vinegar
- 3 eggs
- 1 cup coconut milk

DIRECTIONS

1. In a bowl mix the quinoa, pumpkin seeds, oats and barley
2. Add vinegar and water and stir and allow to soak for 12 hours

3. Heat the oven to 325

4. In a bowl mix coconut oil, maple syrup, eggs and coconut milk

5. Pour the mixture over the soaked grains and stir

6. In a skillet toss the fenugreek and fennel for 2-3 minutes

7. Transfer to the mixing bowl and pour the mixture into a baking dish

8. Bake for 45-50 minutes and remove when golden brown

9. Serve with yogurt or maple syrup

PUMPKIN SPICE GRANOLA

Serves: *4*

Prep Time: *10* Minutes

Cook Time: *30* Minutes

Total Time: *40* Minutes

INGREDIENTS

- 3 cups oats
- 1 cup water
- ¼ cup ghee
- ¼ cup butter
- ¼ cup raisins
- ½ shredded coconut
- ¼ cup yogurt
- ¼ cup pumpkin seeds
- 1 cup nuts
- 1 cup pumpkin puree
- 1 tsp cinnamon powder
- ¼ tsp ginger powder
- ¼ tsp clove powder
- ¼ tsp salt

DIRECTIONS

1. Pour the water over the oats and mix, add yogurt and mix, cover and allow to soak overnight (12 h)

2. In a food processor place the seeds, nuts and blend

3. Add the mixture to the soaked oats

4. In another bowl mix all the ingredients with the pumpkin puree

5. Spread the mixture onto parchment paper lined baking sheets until dry and crispy

6. Remove and serve

PUMPKIN PIE PORRIDGE

Serves: *2*

Prep Time: *10* Minutes

Cook Time: *50* Minutes

Total Time: *60* Minutes

INGREDIENTS

- 1 pie pumpkin
- ½ tsp cloves
- 1 tsp salt
- ¼ cup honey
- 1 cup coconut milk
- 1 tsp cinnamon
- 2 tsp ginger

DIRECTIONS

1. Preheat oven to 325 F
2. Cut pumpkin in half and place the halves in a baking dish
3. Place in the oven and bake for 45 minutes
4. The flesh of the pumpkin blend until smooth and add coconut milk and honey
5. Pour the mixture over the pumpkin and serve

EGGS AND SPINACH

Serves: **4**

Prep Time: **5**   Minutes

Cook Time: **10**   Minutes

Total Time: **15**   Minutes

INGREDIENTS

- 1 ½ tsp chilli flakes
- 4 eggs
- 3 ½ oz spinach
- 1 lb tomatoes

DIRECTIONS

1. Wilt the spinach
2. Squeeze the excess water out
3. Divide among 4 bowls
4. Mix the tomatoes with the seasoning and chilli flakes
5. Add to the spinach bowls
6. Crack an egg into each bowl and bake for about 15 minutes in the preheated oven at 365F

MORNING SAUSAGE

Serves: *4*

Prep Time: *15*   Minutes

Cook Time: *35*   Minutes

Total Time: *50*   Minutes

INGREDIENTS

- 1 lb ground chicken
- 1 ½ tsp smoked paprika
- ½ tsp salt
- 1 ½ tsp rubbed sage
- 1/3 tsp white pepper
- 1/3 tsp thyme
- 1/5 tsp nutmeg
- 1 ½ tbs olive oil

DIRECTIONS

1. Mix the sage, ground meet, paprika, white pepper, nutmeg, thyme and salt
2. Form patties and place them on a baking sheet
3. Fry the patties in hot oil until brown on both sides
4. Serve immediately

BREAKFAST TACO

Serves: **2**

Prep Time: **10** Minutes

Cook Time: **20** Minutes

Total Time: **30** Minutes

INGREDIENTS

- ¼ cup onion
- 1/3 cup green pepper
- 2 tsp sage
- Corn tortillas
- 1 lb turkey
- 1 tsp thyme
- 4 cups eggs
- 2 lb hash browns

DIRECTIONS

1. Mix hash browns and oil, then spread on a baking pan
2. Bake for about 20 minutes until browned
3. Scramble the eggs with onions and peppers
4. Combine the sage and thyme together
5. Fill a tortilla with ½ cup mixture, then microwave for about 15 seconds
6. Serve immediately

STUFFED POTATOES

Serves: *6*

Prep Time: *10*   Minutes

Cook Time: *20*   Minutes

Total Time: *30*   Minutes

INGREDIENTS

- 3 potatoes
- 1/3 cup scallions
- 3 eggs
- 1/3 tsp salt
- 3 tbs butter
- 1/3 tsp pepper
- ½ cup cheese
- ½ cup red pepper

DIRECTIONS

1. Prick potatoes with a fork and microwave for a few minutes until tender
2. Cut the potatoes lengthwise and scoop out the flesh
3. Cook the bell pepper, scallions and chopped potato flesh in melted butter for about 3 minutes
4. Add eggs, salt and pepper and cook 2 more minutes
5. Remove from heat and fold in the cheese

6. **Stuff each potato half with the mixture, allow to cool and wrap with foil**

7. **Refrigerate overnight**

8. **Cook for about 10 minutes turning once**

9. **Serve immediately**

AVOCADO TOAST

Serves: *2*

Prep Time: *5*   Minutes

Cook Time: *5*   Minutes

Total Time: *10*   Minutes

INGREDIENTS

Pesto:

- 1 ½ tbs olive oil
- 1 tbs hot water
- 1/8 tsp black pepper
- ¼ tsp garlic powder
- 1/3 cup basil leaves
- ¼ cup walnuts
- 1 lemon

Toast:

- 1/3 tsp black pepper
- 2 tsp olive oil
- 4 slices bread
- 1 avocado

DIRECTIONS

1. Place the pesto ingredients into a food processor and pulse until smooth
2. Toast the bread

3. Divide the avocado slices

4. Spread pesto over avocado, then drizzle with lemon juice and olive oil

5. Serve immediately

MORNING BAKE

Serves: **12**
Prep Time: **10**   Minutes

Cook Time: **30**   Minutes

Total Time: **40**   Minutes

INGREDIENTS

- 4 eggs
- 3 cups hash brown
- 12 oz turkey sausage
- 1 bell pepper
- 1 cup cheese
- 2 cups milk
- 1 onion
- ½ tsp salt
- ¼ tsp black pepper

DIRECTIONS

1. Cook the onion, pepper and sausage until done
2. Stir together with frozen potatoes and ½ cup cheese, then place into a baking dish
3. Mix together milk, pepper, salt and eggs and pour over
4. Bake uncovered for about 30 minutes
5. Sprinkle with cheese and bake 2 more minutes

HAM OMELETTE

Serves: **2**

Prep Time: **10** Minutes

Cook Time: **20** Minutes

Total Time: **30** Minutes

INGREDIENTS

- 4 eggs
- 1 tbs paprika
- 2 tbs olive oil
- ½ tbs onion powder
- ½ cup onion
- 1/3 cup ham
- ½ cup red pepper
- ½ tbs garlic powder

DIRECTIONS

1. Sauté the onion in hot oil
2. Add in the red pepper and sauté until roasted on edges
3. Add ham and paprika and cook 2 more minutes
4. Whisk together the eggs in a bowl
5. Scramble the eggs in hot oil in another skillet
6. Sprinkle with onion and garlic powder
7. Place the ham mixture on one half of the omelette and fold it

QUICHE CUPS

Serves: *8*
Prep Time: *10*   Minutes

Cook Time: *30*   Minutes

Total Time: *40*   Minutes

INGREDIENTS

- 10 oz broccoli
- 2 drops hot sauce
- 1/3 tsp black pepper
- 4 eggs
- 1 cup cheese
- ½ cup bell peppers
- 1 green onion

DIRECTIONS

1. Squeeze the vegetables dry
2. Blend the ingredients together using a food processor
3. Divide among a lined muffin pan
4. Bake for about 30 minutes
5. Allow to cool, then serve

CHICKEN SAUSAGE

Serves: *4*

Prep Time: *5*   Minutes

Cook Time: *10*   Minutes

Total Time: *15*   Minutes

INGREDIENTS

- ½ tsp red pepper flakes
- 1 ½ tsp maple syrup
- 3 tsp olive oil
- 1 ½ tsp sage
- 1 ½ tsp garlic powder
- 1 ½ tsp black pepper
- 1 lb. ground chicken

DIRECTIONS

1. Mix everything together except for the oil
2. Form patties from the mixture
3. Cook the patties in hot oil until cooked through
4. Serve immediately

BURRITO BOWL

Serves: *4*

Prep Time: *10*   Minutes

Cook Time: *15*   Minutes

Total Time: *25*   Minutes

INGREDIENTS

- 2 tbs olive oil
- ½ cup almond milk
- 2 tbs shallot
- 1 cup red pepper
- 1/3 cup salsa
- 2 eggs
- 2 egg whites
- ½ cup onion
- 2 avocados
- 15 oz pinto beans
- 2 tsp cumin
- 1 cup cherry tomatoes

DIRECTIONS

1. Sauté the onion until soft
2. Add the red peppers and cook until they are also soft

3. Add chili powder, pinto beans and cumin, cook a little more, then cover and turn the heat off

4. Chop the tomatoes and avocados

5. Combine ½ chopped avocado, shallot, salsa and almond milk in a food processor

6. Pulse until combined

7. Scramble the eggs and egg whites

8. Divide the bean mixture into bowls, top with avocado, tomatoes, eggs and drizzle with avocado sauce

9. Serve immediately

HAZELNUT TART

Serves: **6-8**

Prep Time: **25**   Minutes

Cook Time: **25**   Minutes

Total Time: **50**   Minutes

INGREDIENTS

- **pastry sheets**
- **3 oz. brown sugar**
- **¼ lb. hazelnuts**
- **100 ml double cream**
- **2 tablespoons syrup**
- **¼ lb. dark chocolate**
- **2 oz. butter**

DIRECTIONS

1. **Preheat oven to 400 F, unfold pastry sheets and place them on a baking sheet**
2. **Toss together all ingredients together and mix well**
3. **Spread mixture in a single layer on the pastry sheets**
4. **Before baking decorate with your desired fruits**
5. **Bake at 400 F for 22-25 minutes or until golden brown**
6. **When ready remove from the oven and serve**

PEAR TART

Serves: **6-8**

Prep Time: **25**   Minutes

Cook Time: **25**   Minutes

Total Time: **50**   Minutes

INGREDIENTS

- 1 lb. pears
- 2 oz. brown sugar
- ½ lb. flaked almonds
- ¼ lb. porridge oat
- 2 oz. flour
- ¼ lb. almonds
- pastry sheets
- 2 tablespoons syrup

DIRECTIONS

1. **Preheat oven to 400 F, unfold pastry sheets and place them on a baking sheet**
2. **Toss together all ingredients together and mix well**
3. **Spread mixture in a single layer on the pastry sheets**
4. **Before baking decorate with your desired fruits**
5. **Bake at 400 F for 22-25 minutes or until golden brown**
6. **When ready remove from the oven and serve**

PIE RECIPES

PEACH PECAN PIE

Serves: *8-12*

Prep Time: *15*   Minutes

Cook Time: *35*   Minutes

Total Time: *50*   Minutes

INGREDIENTS

- 4-5 cups peaches
- 1 tablespoon preserves
- 1 cup sugar
- 4 small egg yolks
- ¼ cup flour
- 1 tsp vanilla extract

DIRECTIONS

1. Line a pie plate or pie form with pastry and cover the edges of the plate depending on your preference
2. In a bowl combine all pie ingredients together and mix well
3. Pour the mixture over the pastry
4. Bake at 400-425 F for 25-30 minutes or until golden brown
5. When ready remove from the oven and let it rest for 15 minutes

GRAPEFRUIT PIE

Serves: *8-12*

Prep Time: *15*   Minutes

Cook Time: *35*   Minutes

Total Time: *50*   Minutes

INGREDIENTS

- pastry sheets
- 2 cups grapefruit
- 1 cup brown sugar
- ¼ cup flour
- 5-6 egg yolks
- 5 oz. butter

DIRECTIONS

1. Line a pie plate or pie form with pastry and cover the edges of the plate depending on your preference
2. In a bowl combine all pie ingredients together and mix well
3. Pour the mixture over the pastry
4. Bake at 400-425 F for 25-30 minutes or until golden brown
5. When ready remove from the oven and let it rest for 15 minutes

BUTTERFINGER PIE

Serves: **8-12**

Prep Time: **15** Minutes

Cook Time: **35** Minutes

Total Time: **50** Minutes

INGREDIENTS

- pastry sheets
- 1 package cream cheese
- 1 tsp vanilla extract
- ¼ cup peanut butter
- 1 cup powdered sugar (to decorate)
- 2 cups Butterfinger candy bars
- 8 oz whipped topping

DIRECTIONS

1. Line a pie plate or pie form with pastry and cover the edges of the plate depending on your preference
2. In a bowl combine all pie ingredients together and mix well
3. Pour the mixture over the pastry
4. Bake at 400-425 F for 25-30 minutes or until golden brown
5. When ready remove from the oven and let it rest for 15 minutes

SMOOTHIE RECIPES

MACA SMOOTHIE

Serves: *1*

Prep Time: *5*   Minutes

Cook Time: *5*   Minutes

Total Time: *10*   Minutes

INGREDIENTS

- 2 cups hemp milk
- 1 cup ice
- ¼ cup lemon juice
- 2 mangoes
- 1 tablespoon flaxseeds
- 1 tsp maca power
- 1 tsp vanilla extract

DIRECTIONS

1. In a blender place all ingredients and blend until smooth
2. Pour smoothie in a glass and serve

BABY SPINACH SMOOTHIE

Serves: *1*
Prep Time: *5* Minutes

Cook Time: *5* Minutes

Total Time: *10* Minutes

INGREDIENTS

- 1 cup cherry juice
- 1 cup spinach
- 1 cup vanilla yoghurt
- 1 avocado
- 1 cup berries
- 1 tablespoon chia seeds

DIRECTIONS

1. In a blender place all ingredients and blend until smooth
2. Pour smoothie in a glass and serve

SUNRISE SMOOTHIE

Serves: *1*
Prep Time: *5*   Minutes

Cook Time: *5*   Minutes

Total Time: *10*   Minutes

INGREDIENTS

- 1 cup coconut milk
- 1 banana
- ¼ cup lemon juice
- ¼ mango
- 1 tsp almonds
- 1 cup ice

DIRECTIONS

1. In a blender place all ingredients and blend until smooth
2. Pour smoothie in a glass and serve

CUCUMBER SMOOTHIE

Serves: *1*
Prep Time: *5*   Minutes

Cook Time: *5*   Minutes

Total Time: *10* Minutes

INGREDIENTS

- 1 cup vanilla yoghurt
- 1 cup cucumber
- 2 tablespoons dill
- 1 tablespoon basil
- 2 tablespoons mint
- 1 cup ice

DIRECTIONS

1. In a blender place all ingredients and blend until smooth
2. Pour smoothie in a glass and serve

CHERRY SMOOTHIE

Serves: *1*
Prep Time: *5*   Minutes

Cook Time: *5*   Minutes

Total Time: *10*   Minutes

INGREDIENTS

- 1 can cherries
- 2 tablespoons peanut butter
- 1 tablespoon honey
- 1 cup Greek Yoghurt
- 1 cup coconut milk

DIRECTIONS

1. In a blender place all ingredients and blend until smooth
2. Pour smoothie in a glass and serve

CHOCOLATE SMOOTHIE

Serves: *1*
Prep Time: *5*   Minutes

Cook Time: *5*   Minutes

Total Time: *10*   Minutes

INGREDIENTS

- 2 bananas
- 1 cup Greek Yoghurt
- 1 tablespoon honey
- 1 tablespoon cocoa powder
- ½ cup chocolate chips
- ¼ cup almond milk

DIRECTIONS

1. In a blender place all ingredients and blend until smooth
2. Pour smoothie in a glass and serve

TOFU SMOOTHIE

Serves: *1*

Prep Time: *5*   Minutes

Cook Time: *5*   Minutes

Total Time: *10*   Minutes

INGREDIENTS

- 1 cup blueberries
- ¼ cup tofu
- ¼ cup pomegranate juice
- 1 cup ice
- ½ cup agave nectar

DIRECTIONS

1. In a blender place all ingredients and blend until smooth
2. Pour smoothie in a glass and serve

COCONUT SMOOTHIE

Serves: *1*
Prep Time: *5*   Minutes

Cook Time: *5*   Minutes

Total Time: *10*   Minutes

INGREDIENTS

- 1 cup blueberries
- 2 bananas
- 1 cup coconut flakes
- 1 cup coconut milk
- ¼ tsp vanilla essence

DIRECTIONS

1. In a blender place all ingredients and blend until smooth
2. Pour smoothie in a glass and serve

ICE-CREAM RECIPES

SAFFRON ICE-CREAM

Serves: **6-8**

Prep Time: **15** Minutes

Cook Time: **15** Minutes

Total Time: **30** Minutes

INGREDIENTS

- 4 egg yolks
- 1 cup heavy cream
- 1 cup milk
- ½ cup brown sugar
- 1 tsp saffron
- 1 tsp vanilla extract

DIRECTIONS

1. In a saucepan whisk together all ingredients
2. Mix until bubbly
3. Strain into a bowl and cool
4. Whisk in favorite fruits and mix well
5. Cover and refrigerate for 2-3 hours
6. Pour mixture in the ice-cream maker and follow manufacturer instructions
7. Serve when ready

PISTACHIOS ICE-CREAM

Serves: **6-8**

Prep Time: **15**   Minutes

Cook Time: **15**   Minutes

Total Time: **30**   Minutes

INGREDIENTS

- **4 egg yolks**
- **1 cup heavy cream**
- **1 cup milk**
- **1 cup sugar**
- **1 vanilla bean**
- **1 tsp almond extract**
- **1 cup cherries**
- **½ cup pistachios**

DIRECTIONS

1. **In a saucepan whisk together all ingredients**
2. **Mix until bubbly**
3. **Strain into a bowl and cool**
4. **Whisk in favorite fruits and mix well**
5. **Cover and refrigerate for 2-3 hours**
6. **Pour mixture in the ice-cream maker and follow manufacturer instructions**

THIRD COOKBOOK

BLUEBERRY PANCAKES

Serves: **4**

Prep Time: **10** Minutes

Cook Time: **20** Minutes

Total Time: **30** Minutes

INGREDIENTS

- 1 cup whole wheat flour
- ¼ tsp baking soda
- ¼ tsp baking powder
- 1 cup blueberries
- 2 eggs
- 1 cup milk

DIRECTIONS

1. In a bowl combine all ingredients together and mix well
2. In a skillet heat olive oil
3. Pour ¼ of the batter and cook each pancake for 1-2 minutes per side
4. When ready remove from heat and serve

MULBERRIES PANCAKES

Serves: **4**

Prep Time: **10**   Minutes

Cook Time: **30**   Minutes

Total Time: **40**   Minutes

INGREDIENTS

- 1 cup whole wheat flour
- ¼ tsp baking soda
- ¼ tsp baking powder
- 1 cup mulberries
- 2 eggs
- 1 cup milk

DIRECTIONS

1. In a bowl combine all ingredients together and mix well
2. In a skillet heat olive oil
3. Pour ¼ of the batter and cook each pancake for 1-2 minutes per side
4. When ready remove from heat and serve

BANANA PANCAKES

Serves: **4**

Prep Time: **10** Minutes

Cook Time: **20** Minutes

Total Time: **30** Minutes

INGREDIENTS

- 1 cup whole wheat flour
- ¼ tsp baking soda
- ¼ tsp baking powder
- 1 cup mashed banana
- 2 eggs
- 1 cup milk

DIRECTIONS

1. In a bowl combine all ingredients together and mix well
2. In a skillet heat olive oil
3. Pour ¼ of the batter and cook each pancake for 1-2 minutes per side
4. When ready remove from heat and serve

NECTARINE PANCAKES

Serves: *4*
Prep Time: *10*   Minutes

Cook Time: *20*   Minutes

Total Time: *30*   Minutes

INGREDIENTS

- 1 cup whole wheat flour
- ¼ tsp baking soda
- ¼ tsp baking powder
- 1 cup nectarines
- 2 eggs
- 1 cup milk

DIRECTIONS

1. In a bowl combine all ingredients together and mix well
2. In a skillet heat olive oil
3. Pour ¼ of the batter and cook each pancake for 1-2 minutes per side
4. When ready remove from heat and serve

PANCAKES

Serves: **4**

Prep Time: **10** Minutes

Cook Time: **30** Minutes

Total Time: **40** Minutes

INGREDIENTS

- 1 cup whole wheat flour
- ¼ tsp baking soda
- ¼ tsp baking powder
- 2 eggs
- 1 cup milk

DIRECTIONS

1. In a bowl combine all ingredients together and mix well
2. In a skillet heat olive oil
3. Pour ¼ of the batter and cook each pancake for 1-2 minutes per side
4. When ready remove from heat and serve

BLUEBERRY MUFFINS

Serves: *8-12*

Prep Time: *10*   Minutes

Cook Time: *20*   Minutes

Total Time: *30*   Minutes

INGREDIENTS

- 2 eggs
- 1 tablespoon olive oil
- 1 cup milk
- 2 cups whole wheat flour
- 1 tsp baking soda
- ¼ tsp baking soda
- 1 tsp cinnamon
- 1 cup blueberries

DIRECTIONS

1. In a bowl combine all wet ingredients
2. In another bowl combine all dry ingredients
3. Combine wet and dry ingredients together
4. Fold in blueberries and mix well
5. Pour mixture into 8-12 prepared muffin cups, fill 2/3 of the cups
6. Bake for 18-20 minutes at 375 F

KUMQUAT MUFFINS

Serves: *8-12*

Prep Time: *10*   Minutes

Cook Time: *20*   Minutes

Total Time: *30*   Minutes

INGREDIENTS

- 2 eggs
- 1 tablespoon olive oil
- 1 cup milk
- 2 cups whole wheat flour
- 1 tsp baking soda
- ¼ tsp baking soda
- 1 tsp cinnamon
- 1 cup kumquat

DIRECTIONS

1. In a bowl combine all wet ingredients
2. In another bowl combine all dry ingredients
3. Combine wet and dry ingredients together
4. Pour mixture into 8-12 prepared muffin cups, fill 2/3 of the cups
5. Bake for 18-20 minutes at 375 F
6. When ready remove from the oven and serve

CHOCOLATE MUFFINS

Serves: *8-12*

Prep Time: *10*   Minutes

Cook Time: *20*   Minutes

Total Time: *30*   Minutes

INGREDIENTS

- 2 eggs
- 1 tablespoon olive oil
- 1 cup milk
- 2 cups whole wheat flour
- 1 tsp baking soda
- ¼ tsp baking soda
- 1 tsp cinnamon
- 1 cup chocolate chips

DIRECTIONS

1. In a bowl combine all wet ingredients
2. In another bowl combine all dry ingredients
3. Combine wet and dry ingredients together
4. Fold in chocolate chips and mix well
5. Pour mixture into 8-12 prepared muffin cups, fill 2/3 of the cups
6. Bake for 18-20 minutes at 375 F

MUFFINS

Serves: *8-12*

Prep Time: *10*   Minutes

Cook Time: *20*   Minutes

Total Time: *30*   Minutes

INGREDIENTS

- 2 eggs
- 1 tablespoon olive oil
- 1 cup milk
- 2 cups whole wheat flour
- 1 tsp baking soda
- ¼ tsp baking soda
- 1 tsp cinnamon

DIRECTIONS

1. In a bowl combine all wet ingredients
2. In another bowl combine all dry ingredients
3. Combine wet and dry ingredients together
4. Pour mixture into 8-12 prepared muffin cups, fill 2/3 of the cups
5. Bake for 18-20 minutes at 375 F
6. When ready remove from the oven and serve

OMELETTE

Serves: *1*
Prep Time: *5*   Minutes

Cook Time: *10*   Minutes

Total Time: *15*   Minutes

INGREDIENTS

- 2 eggs
- ¼ tsp salt
- ¼ tsp black pepper
- 1 tablespoon olive oil
- ¼ cup cheese
- ¼ tsp basil

DIRECTIONS

1. In a bowl combine all ingredients together and mix well
2. In a skillet heat olive oil and pour the egg mixture
3. Cook for 1-2 minutes per side
4. When ready remove omelette from the skillet and serve

CARROT OMELETTE

Serves: *1*
Prep Time: *5*   Minutes

Cook Time: *10*   Minutes

Total Time: *15*   Minutes

INGREDIENTS

- 2 eggs
- ¼ tsp salt
- ¼ tsp black pepper
- 1 tablespoon olive oil
- ¼ cup cheese
- ¼ tsp basil
- 1 cup carrot

DIRECTIONS

1. In a bowl combine all ingredients together and mix well
2. In a skillet heat olive oil and pour the egg mixture
3. Cook for 1-2 minutes per side
4. When ready remove omelette from the skillet and serve

ONION OMELETTE

Serves: *1*
Prep Time: *5*   Minutes

Cook Time: *10*   Minutes

Total Time: *15*   Minutes

INGREDIENTS

- 2 eggs
- ¼ tsp salt
- ¼ tsp black pepper
- 1 tablespoon olive oil
- ¼ cup cheese
- ¼ tsp basil
- 1 cup red onion

DIRECTIONS

1. In a bowl combine all ingredients together and mix well
2. In a skillet heat olive oil and pour the egg mixture
3. Cook for 1-2 minutes per side
4. When ready remove omelette from the skillet and serve

BROCCOLI OMELETTE

Serves: *1*

Prep Time: *5*   Minutes

Cook Time: *10* Minutes

Total Time: *15* Minutes

INGREDIENTS

- 2 eggs
- ¼ tsp salt
- ¼ tsp black pepper
- 1 tablespoon olive oil
- ¼ cup cheese
- ¼ tsp basil
- 1 cup broccoli

DIRECTIONS

1. In a bowl combine all ingredients together and mix well
2. In a skillet heat olive oil and pour the egg mixture
3. Cook for 1-2 minutes per side
4. When ready remove omelette from the skillet and serve

BEETS OMELETTE

Serves: *1*

Prep Time: *5*   Minutes

Cook Time: *10*   Minutes

Total Time: *15*   Minutes

INGREDIENTS

- 2 eggs
- ¼ tsp salt
- ¼ tsp black pepper
- 1 tablespoon olive oil
- ¼ cup cheese
- ¼ tsp basil
- 1 cup beets

DIRECTIONS

1. In a bowl combine all ingredients together and mix well
2. In a skillet heat olive oil and pour the egg mixture
3. Cook for 1-2 minutes per side
4. When ready remove omelette from the skillet and serve

BREAKFAST GRANOLA

Serves: 2

Prep Time: 5   Minutes

Cook Time: 30   Minutes

Total Time: 35   Minutes

INGREDIENTS

- 1 tsp vanilla extract
- 1 tablespoon honey
- 1 lb. rolled oats
- 2 tablespoons sesame seeds
- ¼ lb. almonds
- ¼ lb. berries

DIRECTIONS

1. Preheat the oven to 325 F
2. Spread the granola onto a baking sheet
3. Bake for 12-15 minutes, remove and mix everything
4. Bake for another 12-15 minutes or until slightly brown
5. When ready remove from the oven and serve

Serves: **1**

Prep Time: **5**   Minutes

Cook Time: **5**   Minutes

Total Time: **10**   Minutes

INGREDIENTS

- ½ cup dried raisins
- ½ cup dried pecans
- ¼ cup almonds
- 1 cup coconut milk
- 1 tsp cinnamon

DIRECTIONS

1. In a bowl combine all ingredients together
2. Serve with milk

SAUSAGE BREAKFAST SANDWICH

Serves: 2

Prep Time: 5   Minutes

Cook Time: 15   Minutes

Total Time: 20   Minutes

INGREDIENTS

- ¼ cup egg substitute
- 1 muffin
- 1 turkey sausage patty
- 1 tablespoon cheddar cheese

DIRECTIONS

1. In a skillet pour egg and cook on low heat
2. Place turkey sausage patty in a pan and cook for 4-5 minutes per side
3. On a toasted muffin place the cooked egg, top with a sausage patty and cheddar cheese
4. Serve when ready

Serves: *8-12*

Prep Time: *10*   Minutes

Cook Time: *20*   Minutes

Total Time: *30*   Minutes

INGREDIENTS

- 2 eggs
- 1 tablespoon olive oil
- 1 cup milk
- 2 cups whole wheat flour
- 1 tsp baking soda
- ¼ tsp baking soda
- 1 tsp cinnamon
- 1 cup strawberries

DIRECTIONS

1. In a bowl combine all wet ingredients
2. In another bowl combine all dry ingredients
3. Combine wet and dry ingredients together
4. Pour mixture into 8-12 prepared muffin cups, fill 2/3 of the cups
5. Bake for 18-20 minutes at 375 F
6. When ready remove from the oven and serve

BREAKFAST COOKIES

Serves: *8-12*

Prep Time: *5*   Minutes

Cook Time: *15*   Minutes

Total Time: *20*   Minutes

INGREDIENTS

- 1 cup rolled oats
- ¼ cup applesauce
- ½ tsp vanilla extract
- 3 tablespoons chocolate chips
- 2 tablespoons dried fruits
- 1 tsp cinnamon

DIRECTIONS

1. Preheat the oven to 325 F
2. In a bowl combine all ingredients together and mix well
3. Scoop cookies using an ice cream scoop
4. Place cookies onto a prepared baking sheet
5. Place in the oven for 12-15 minutes or until the cookies are done
6. When ready remove from the oven and serve

GRAPEFRUIT PIE

Serves: *8-12*

Prep Time: *15*   Minutes

Cook Time: *35*   Minutes

Total Time: *50*   Minutes

INGREDIENTS

- pastry sheets
- 2 cups grapefruit
- 1 cup brown sugar
- ¼ cup flour
- 5-6 egg yolks
- 5 oz. butter

DIRECTIONS

1. Line a pie plate or pie form with pastry and cover the edges of the plate depending on your preference
2. In a bowl combine all pie ingredients together and mix well
3. Pour the mixture over the pastry
4. Bake at 400-425 F for 25-30 minutes or until golden brown
5. When ready remove from the oven and let it rest for 15 minutes

Serves: *8-12*

Prep Time: *15*   Minutes

Cook Time: *35*   Minutes

Total Time: *50*   Minutes

INGREDIENTS

- pastry sheets
- 1 package cream cheese
- 1 tsp vanilla extract
- ¼ cup peanut butter
- 1 cup powdered sugar (to decorate)
- 2 cups Butterfinger candy bars
- 8 oz whipped topping

DIRECTIONS

1. Line a pie plate or pie form with pastry and cover the edges of the plate depending on your preference
2. In a bowl combine all pie ingredients together and mix well
3. Pour the mixture over the pastry
4. Bake at 400-425 F for 25-30 minutes or until golden brown
5. When ready remove from the oven and let it rest for 15 minutes

STRAWBERRY PIE

Serves: **8-12**

Prep Time: **15**   Minutes

Cook Time: **35**   Minutes

Total Time: **50**   Minutes

INGREDIENTS

- pastry sheets
- 1,5 lb. strawberries
- 1 cup powdered sugar
- 2 tablespoons cornstarch
- 1 tablespoon lime juice
- 1 tsp vanilla extract
- 2 eggs
- 2 tablespoons butter

DIRECTIONS

1. Line a pie plate or pie form with pastry and cover the edges of the plate depending on your preference
2. In a bowl combine all pie ingredients together and mix well
3. Pour the mixture over the pastry
4. Bake at 400-425 F for 25-30 minutes or until golden brown
5. When ready remove from the oven and let it rest for 15 minutes

BLUEBERRY PIE

Serves: *8-12*

Prep Time: *15*   Minutes

Cook Time: *35*   Minutes

Total Time: *50*   Minutes

INGREDIENTS

- pastry sheets
- ¼ tsp lavender
- 1 cup brown sugar
- 4-5 cups blueberries
- 1 tablespoon lemon juice
- 1 cup almonds
- 2 tablespoons butter

DIRECTIONS

1. Line a pie plate or pie form with pastry and cover the edges of the plate depending on your preference
2. In a bowl combine all pie ingredients together and mix well
3. Pour the mixture over the pastry
4. Bake at 400-425 F for 25-30 minutes or until golden brown
5. When ready remove from the oven and let it rest for 15 minutes

PUMPKIN PIE

Serves: *8-12*
Prep Time: *15*   Minutes

Cook Time: *35*   Minutes

Total Time: *50*   Minutes

INGREDIENTS

- pastry sheets
- 1 cup buttermilk
- 1 can pumpkin
- 1 cup sugar
- 1 tsp cinnamon
- 1 tsp vanilla extract
- 2 eggs

DIRECTIONS

1. Line a pie plate or pie form with pastry and cover the edges of the plate depending on your preference
2. In a bowl combine all pie ingredients together and mix well
3. Pour the mixture over the pastry
4. Bake at 400-425 F for 25-30 minutes or until golden brown
5. When ready remove from the oven and let it rest for 15 minutes

RICOTTA ICE-CREAM

Serves: *6-8*

Prep Time: *15*   Minutes

Cook Time: *15*   Minutes

Total Time: *30*   Minutes

INGREDIENTS

- 1 cup almonds
- 1-pint vanilla ice cream
- 2 cups ricotta cheese
- 1 cup honey

DIRECTIONS

1. In a saucepan whisk together all ingredients
2. Mix until bubbly
3. Strain into a bowl and cool
4. Whisk in favorite fruits and mix well
5. Cover and refrigerate for 2-3 hours
6. Pour mixture in the ice-cream maker and follow manufacturer instructions
7. Serve when ready

SAFFRON ICE-CREAM

Serves: **6-8**

Prep Time: **15**   Minutes

Cook Time: **15**   Minutes

Total Time: **30**   Minutes

INGREDIENTS

- 4 egg yolks
- 1 cup heavy cream
- 1 cup milk
- ½ cup brown sugar
- 1 tsp saffron
- 1 tsp vanilla extract

DIRECTIONS

1. In a saucepan whisk together all ingredients
2. Mix until bubbly
3. Strain into a bowl and cool
4. Whisk in favorite fruits and mix well
5. Cover and refrigerate for 2-3 hours
6. Pour mixture in the ice-cream maker and follow manufacturer instructions
7. Serve when ready

PISTACHIOS ICE-CREAM

Serves: **6-8**

Prep Time: **15**   Minutes

Cook Time: **15**   Minutes

Total Time: **30**   Minutes

INGREDIENTS

- 4 egg yolks
- 1 cup heavy cream
- 1 cup milk
- 1 cup sugar
- 1 vanilla bean
- 1 tsp almond extract
- 1 cup cherries
- ½ cup pistachios

DIRECTIONS

1. In a saucepan whisk together all ingredients
2. Mix until bubbly
3. Strain into a bowl and cool
4. Whisk in favorite fruits and mix well
5. Cover and refrigerate for 2-3 hours
6. Pour mixture in the ice-cream maker and follow manufacturer instructions

VANILLA ICE-CREAM

Serves: *6-8*

Prep Time: *15* Minutes

Cook Time: *15* Minutes

Total Time: *30* Minutes

INGREDIENTS

- 1 cup milk
- 1 tablespoon cornstarch
- 1 oz. cream cheese
- 1 cup heavy cream
- 1 cup brown sugar
- 1 tablespoon corn syrup
- 1 vanilla bean

DIRECTIONS

1. In a saucepan whisk together all ingredients
2. Mix until bubbly
3. Strain into a bowl and cool
4. Whisk in favorite fruits and mix well
5. Cover and refrigerate for 2-3 hours
6. Pour mixture in the ice-cream maker and follow manufacturer instructions
7. Serve when ready

COFFE ICE-CREAM

Serves: **6-8**

Prep Time: **15**   Minutes

Cook Time: **15**   Minutes

Total Time: **30**   Minutes

INGREDIENTS

- 4 egg yolks
- 1 cup black coffee
- 2 cups heavy cream
- 1 cup half-and-half
- 1 cup brown sugar
- 1 tsp vanilla extract

DIRECTIONS

1. In a saucepan whisk together all ingredients
2. Mix until bubbly
3. Strain into a bowl and cool
4. Whisk in favorite fruits and mix well
5. Cover and refrigerate for 2-3 hours
6. Pour mixture in the ice-cream maker and follow manufacturer instructions
7. Serve when ready

STRAWBERRY ICE-CREAM

Serves: **6-8**

Prep Time: **15**   Minutes

Cook Time: **15**   Minutes

Total Time: **30**   Minutes

INGREDIENTS

- 1 lb. strawberries
- ½ cup sugar
- 1 tablespoon vanilla extract
- 1 cup heavy cram
- 1-pint vanilla

DIRECTIONS

1. In a saucepan whisk together all ingredients
2. Mix until bubbly
3. Strain into a bowl and cool
4. Whisk in favorite fruits and mix well
5. Cover and refrigerate for 2-3 hours
6. Pour mixture in the ice-cream maker and follow manufacturer instructions
7. Serve when ready

CREAMSICLE SMOOTHIE

Serves: **1**

Prep Time: **5** Minutes

Cook Time: **5** Minutes

Total Time: **10** Minutes

INGREDIENTS

- 2 cups mango
- 1 carrot
- 1 tablespoon apple cider vinegar
- 1 tsp lemon juice
- 1 cup coconut milk
- 1 tsp honey

DIRECTIONS

1. In a blender place all ingredients and blend until smooth
2. Pour smoothie in a glass and serve

BUTTERMILK SMOOTHIE

Serves: **1**

Prep Time: **5**   Minutes

Cook Time: **5**   Minutes

Total Time: **10** Minutes

INGREDIENTS

- 1 cup strawberries
- 1 cup buttermilk
- 1 cup ice
- 1 tsp honey
- 1 tsp agave syrup

DIRECTIONS

1. In a blender place all ingredients and blend until smooth
2. Pour smoothie in a glass and serve

Serves: *1*
Prep Time: 5   Minutes

Cook Time: 5   Minutes

Total Time: *10*   Minutes

INGREDIENTS

- 1 banana
- 1 cup pineapple
- ¼ cup parsley
- 1 tsp chia seeds
- 1 cup ice

DIRECTIONS

1. In a blender place all ingredients and blend until smooth
2. Pour smoothie in a glass and serve

POMEGRANATE SMOOTHIE

Serves: *1*
Prep Time: *5*   Minutes

Cook Time: *5*   Minutes

Total Time: *10*   Minutes

INGREDIENTS

- 1 cup pomegranate juice
- ¼ cup vanilla yogurt
- 3 cooked beets
- ¼ cup grapefruit juice
- 1 tablespoon honey
- 1 cup ice

DIRECTIONS

1. In a blender place all ingredients and blend until smooth
2. Pour smoothie in a glass and serve

CASHEW SMOOTHIE

Serves: *1*
Prep Time: 5   Minutes

Cook Time: 5   Minutes

Total Time: *10*   Minutes

INGREDIENTS

- 1 cup cashew milk
- 1 cup vanilla yogurt
- 1 banana
- 1 cup pumpkin puree
- 1 cup ice

DIRECTIONS

1. In a blender place all ingredients and blend until smooth
2. Pour smoothie in a glass and serve

CELERY SMOOTHIE

Serves: *1*
Prep Time: **5**   Minutes

Cook Time: **5**   Minutes

Total Time: **10** Minutes

INGREDIENTS

- 1 cup pineapple
- 1 cup cucumber
- 1 cup celery
- 1 tablespoon basil
- 1 tsp lemon juice
- 1 cup ice

DIRECTIONS

1. In a blender place all ingredients and blend until smooth
2. Pour smoothie in a glass and serve

COCO SMOOTHIE

Serves: *1*

Prep Time: **5**   Minutes

Cook Time: **5**   Minutes

Total Time: **10**   Minutes

INGREDIENTS

- 1 cup coconut milk
- 1 cup coconut yogurt
- 1 banana
- ½ cup chocolate chips
- 1 cup ice
- 1 pinch cinnamon

DIRECTIONS

1. In a blender place all ingredients and blend until smooth
2. Pour smoothie in a glass and serve

Serves: **1**

Prep Time: **5** Minutes

Cook Time: **5** Minutes

Total Time: **10** Minutes

INGREDIENTS

- 1 cup almond milk
- 1 cup vanilla yogurt
- 1 cup cranberries
- 1 pear
- 1 tablespoon honey
- 1 cup ice

DIRECTIONS

1. In a blender place all ingredients and blend until smooth
2. Pour smoothie in a glass and serve

GINGER SMOOTHIE

Serves: *1*

Prep Time: 5   Minutes

Cook Time: 5   Minutes

Total Time: *10*   Minutes

INGREDIENTS

- 1 cup buttermilk
- 1/2 cup yogurt
- 1-inch ginger
- 1 tablespoon agave syrup
- 1 cup ice

DIRECTIONS

1. In a blender place all ingredients and blend until smooth
2. Pour smoothie in a glass and serve

DATE SMOOTHIE

Serves: **1**

Prep Time: **5** Minutes

Cook Time: **5** Minutes

Total Time: **10** Minutes

INGREDIENTS

- ½ cup dates
- 1 cup almond milk
- 1 pinch cinnamon
- 1 cup ice
- ¼ cup pomegranate juice

DIRECTIONS

1. In a blender place all ingredients and blend until smooth
2. Pour smoothie in a glass and serve

THANK YOU FOR READING THIS BOOK!

CPSIA information can be obtained
at www.ICGtesting.com
Printed in the USA
BVHW031012150321
602551BV00004B/243